CONTROL YOUR WEIGHT

Francine Boucher   **Robert Pauzé**

CONTROL YOUR WEIGHT

- Without dieting
- In 10 weeks
- Permanently

**A guide to self-managing
your eating behavior**

S.O.C.P.

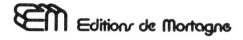 Editions de Mortagne

Published by :
Editions de Mortagne
250, Industrial Boulevard
Boucherville (Quebec)
J4B 2X4
Tel. : (514) 641-2387

Consulting Publisher :
S.O.C.P.
Université de Montréal
2101, Edouard Montpetit Boulevard
Montreal, Quebec
H3C 3J7

Translation :
Blanche Hodder

Cover Illustration :
Clic Communications

Legal deposit :
National Library of Canada
National Library of Quebec
October 1989

ISBN : 2-89074-904-5

1 2 3 4 - 89 - 92 91 90 89

Printed in Canada

This program was created by the Psychological Guidance and Consultation Service of the University of Montreal in collaboration with the Health Service.

The University of Montreal's Psychological Guidance and Consultation Service, with 11 practising psychologists who are members of recognized professional organizations, offers university students and staff, as well as the general public, a complete range of psychological services.

S.O.C.P.
2101, boul. Édouard-Montpetit
Montréal, H3C 3J7

Tél. : (514) 343-6853.

TABLE OF CONTENTS

INTRODUCTION

Another weight-control plan! If you're like most overweight people, this is not the first program you've come across and no doubt you're wondering if these authors will urge you to eat cottage cheese or grapefruit or just half-starve yourself for a couple of months.

Your problem worries you enough to make you read this book and perhaps you hope that this time the "experts" will offer you a suitable solution.

You want to lose weight. You remember yesterday's excesses or you're thinking of an upcoming social affair. Your motivation is currently on the rise but, at the same time, you're doubtful, you're hesitant. You know from experience with previous diets that one day or the next you'll weaken and, little by little, you'll regain the weight you lost and maybe even a few pounds extra.

Your doubts are certainly justified; this story repeats itself thousands of times a year. Do you know that only 5% to 7% of people enrolled in a weight-control program maintain their weight loss after 6 months or a year?

Diets rarely succeed at permanently solving weight problems. Old habits return when your favorite foods are in front of you and the cycle begins anew.

This guide will not offer you any diet.

"And I can lose weight in spite of everything? I'll keep on losing weight without doing anything?"

If you follow this guide, you will lose weight in spite of everything, but there is something you must do: learn to solve a problem, i.e. put time and energy into redefining it, make a list of solutions, apply them and re-evaluate the situation when changes are called for. So you see, no diet, just a hearty helping of motivation to solve the problem once and for all.

"But," you say, "I don't know why I eat so much" or "I know what the problem is but it doesn't keep me from eating. What I have to do is so boring, so frustrating."

This guide will teach you how to define your problem and how to solve it satisfactorily for you. It will not offer a solution that becomes so frustrating in the long term that you'll want to end the treatment. On the contrary, it offers you the chance to create your own solutions by giving you all the information you need to develop this skill when it comes to food intake.

What are your chances of succeeding at what we recommend? The factors for success are many and complex but three are essential: be motivated, know and effectively practise the process of solving problems and possess a body of knowledge relating to obesity problems.

We will give you the theoretical and technical information you need. Are you motivated? If yes, follow the guide...

A BRIEF BACKGROUND

For a long time, medical science has maintained that obesity is the result of eating too much for the amount of energy you expend. Obesity is the consequence of a positive energy imbalance.

The main methods of treating the problem derive from this theoretical premise; essentially they aim at reducing food consumption through a controlled diet or at increasing energy expenditure through a physical exercise program, or they combine both approaches.

Stunkard (1976), a well-known researcher in the field, sums up the therapeutic results obtained as follows: some overweight patients do not commit themselves to an obesity treatment; among those who do commit themselves, some do not complete the treatment; among those who complete the treatment, some do not lose much weight; among those who lose weight, some put it back on; only 12% of patients lose more than 20 pounds, and only 2% succeed in maintaining this weight loss.

Despite the medical evidence, the prescribed treatment (diet, physical exercise or the two combined) is not followed by the majority of patients. One could say that the overweight person lacks the "willpower" for a strict diet and after several lapses abandons the treatment or, once the treatment is completed, returns to his or her old eating habits and regains the lost weight.

On their side,[1] psychiatry and psychology allege that certain emotional problems underlying the obesity problem push the patient to overeat and thus a diet solves nothing. As the primary treatment step, psychotherapy is advised so that patients can first recognize the psychological factors which cause the problem and then, little by little, take themselves in hand to act more satisfactorily on their lives. The therapeutic results of this approach have not been scientifically collated except in a few cases. Thus, we cannot generalize for the overweight population as a whole. In some cases, the treatment succeeds...and is spaced out over quite a long time period. If traditional psychotherapy is shown to be the only effective treatment, the overweight person cannot hope to reach a comfortable weight until after two, three or more years of intensive sessions.

During the 1960s and 1970s, the problem of obesity was tackled from another angle : the behavioral approach. Researchers (Ferster et al., 1962) developed a new treatment mode based on the psychology of learning. Reports multiplied and during 1972, R. Stuart and B. Davis, in a book entitled, "Slim Chance in a Fat World," reported the best results ever obtained in obesity treatment. The weight-loss curve for the patients treated over a one-year period showed a continuous weight loss. Not just 25% but all of the patients observed lost over 20 pounds. Not 5% but 50% of patients lost more than 40 pounds.

Behavioral therapy is the treatment mode we are offering. The brief description which follows will allow you to judge the effectiveness of such a program for you.

---

1. For an excellent treatment of the subject, see "Eating Disorders, Anorexia Nervosa and the Person Within", Hilde Bruch, Basic Books, New York.

A TREATMENT PROGRAM

The behavioral approach does not hold that an obese person has difficulty controlling his or her weight but rather that the person controls (self-manages) his or her environment in such a way as to put on weight. Perhaps the term self-management is inappropriate, inasmuch as the overweight person often has the impression of lacking control; he or she feels guilty of being too greedy, particularly in cases where the person knows the principles of good nutrition and has sometimes even correctly identified psychological factors which cause overeating.

> **What are the causes of the problem ? Behavior. An overweight person acts in a way that puts on weight. The behavior, which in time becomes a habit, perpetuates the problem.**

DEFINING OBESITY

To understand the treatment properly, let's first dispel some preconceptions about obesity.
1. Obesity is not a hereditary disease ; excess fat in the tissues is not written into the individual genetic code.
2. It is often believed that obesity is a hormonal illness or that it results from a malfunction of the thyroid gland. Research in the health sciences demonstrates that only a tiny percentage of weight problems arise from hormonal dysfunctions.
3. Obesity is not necessarily symptomatic of mental abnormality. One can learn to alter eating behavior without undergoing therapy or undergo therapy without losing weight.
4. Obesity does not result from an innate lack of willpower. It would be too easy to believe that some people are born with this marvelous quality while others are deprived of it forever. Self-control can be developed. You can learn to self-manage your life and, you'll see, your ideas about willpower will soon change.

Obesity is an excess of fatty or adipose tissue in the organism. In small quantities, fat is an energy reserve, a good insulator and an indispensable element in the absorption and use of Vitamins A, D, E and K. In excess, fat causes a number of physical and aesthetic problems. This excess is the result of an energy imbalance between the number of calories absorbed and the number of calories expended. Each time the body's needs are exceeded by 3 500 calories, approximately one pound is added to body weight, whether these calories are in the form of carbohydrates, proteins or fats.

> **The difference between the obese and the non-obese lies principally in their living habits, eating and physical-activity behavior and in their self-management skills.**

If you have already been on a diet, you know better than anyone else what an effort it takes to lose weight. All this effort is aimed at eliminating a symptom : weight. But the problem remains untouched since the causes related to eating habits and energy expenditure are not treated. Although the ultimate goal is weight loss, the program we offer aims first at modifying eating behavior as well as becoming sensitized to physical activity. Therefore, it aims at treating the causes of the problem and not at eliminating the symptom.

Self-managing one's life means defining and solving the problems that come up. Since your present behavior perpetuates the obesity problem, it must be analyzed to discover the stimuli or specific causes that lead you to overeat or to eat fattening foods. The causes revealed will become the target of change strategies for you to test so you can then assess their effectiveness and begin again, if necessary, with a new definition of the situation (new behavioral targets) until a satisfactory solution has been reached.

By learning to self-manage your eating behavior, you'll be able to choose, little by little, the life habits which correspond to your goals. Out with restrictions ; make way for action !

The program

As we mentioned before, success in obesity treatment is not just a question of willpower. The three main factors necessary to the treatment's success are as follows:

1. Acquire certain behavioral and psychological skills.
2. Get information on food intake and energy expenditure.
3. Have the motivation needed to meet the treatment's requirements.

These factors are the structural support of the program so look them over more attentively.

1. Acquire certain behavioral and psychological skills

This guide teaches three major skills with respect to the goal pursued: controlling the eating environment, solving problems and eliminating irrational ideas about the problem of obesity. In this treatment program, you'll find all the relevant information for developing these skills. First, let's look at what they represent in theory.

a) Controlling the eating environment

Eating behavior always takes place in a given environment. Thus your eating behavior will be different if you are with strangers or with friends who like to eat in large quantities, if you are at home or in a restaurant, if you have a lot or a little time to eat, etc. So the external environment has a great deal of influence on the quantity and quality of food consumption.

To learn the effect of the environment on your behavior, we propose that you gather all relevant data about your eating habits. You will enter these observations in a diary: what, when, where, and the events which preceded or followed your behavior. Piece by piece, patterns will emerge and you will learn to control your environment to eliminate problem areas.

The environment is the pastry shop on your way home, the friend who loves to eat, the chocolate in the cupboard...but it's also the habit of eating while watching television or snacking several times a day. The environment is a host of associations which have been established with time between certain events and your eating behavior. Some stimuli have acquired the power to set off eating behavior and others outrightly encourage it. For example, I make a cake to please a friend, who is delighted, and my friend's pleasure makes me feel so good that I do it again.

To weaken the links between external events and problem eating behavior, you must make yourself follow rules which will teach you how to acquire good eating habits and spur you in this direction. For example, the first rule will oblige you always to eat while seated and the second, to eat only in food environments (kitchens, dining rooms, restaurants, etc.). Since these rules are cumulative, two weeks after the program begins, you should at all times be eating while seated in a food environment. These rules will reduce your food consumption and prevent food "attacks" which are otherwise so difficult to avoid or control.

b) Solving the problem

Up to now, we have talked about the process of solving problems (PSP), pointing out that it is an indispensable skill in self-managing your life. Practising problem-solving reflects a responsible, logical and active attitude in the face of daily problems. What is its technique?

Problem-solving is a circular process in six phases. The term "circular" means that, depending on the problem's complexity, it is sometimes necessary to repeat the process several times before arriving at the most appropriate solution. For example, you want a clearer understanding of a text in French. First, you'll need a dictionary and a grammar; you estimate you'll have about five hours of work and you set yourself to the task since you are not yet perfectly bilingual. When the time period ends, you evaluate the situation and see that a third of the work remains to be done. Then you redefine the coordinates of the situation to find a new solution. It becomes a new PSP. Obesity problems are rarely as simple as making a translation. You may have to go through several PSPs before reaching your goal. Here are the six phases. You will learn to put them into practice as the treatment progresses.

1. **Defining the problem:** Gather all data relevant to the target behavior without any preconceived notions or prior interpretation. This step is decisive to your chances of success because a faulty definition of the problem will affect the entire process. The difficulty inherent in this task is easy to recognize, since the definition of the situation varies with the observer. The interpretation system we're offering you will become clear when you have progressed in the program. By adopting it, you will succeed at controlling your behavior.

2. **Listing the solutions:** Find as many solutions as possible to the problem without criticizing or rejecting them. At this step in the process, the quantity of solutions takes precedence over their quality. Creativity is a major trump card here.

3. **Analyzing the solutions:** Appraise the solutions found in terms of their relevance to solving the problem.

4. **Choosing one or more solutions:** Decide on one or several solutions among those which have been evaluated in the preceding step. It is important to choose realistic solutions which can be applied at the chosen moment.

5. **Applying the solution:** First, plan the mode of application (opportune moment, material, time-table, etc.) and second, proceed to applying the solution(s) planned.

6. **Evaluating the solution:** Once the solution has been applied, evaluate its adequacy. As we have already mentioned, a problem is rarely settled once and for all. By accepting the need for progressive steps, you'll succeed at reaching your goal.

c) Controlling irrational ideas

Mahoney and Mahoney (1976) described three types of irrational ideas often expressed by people who want to lose weight : unrealistic goals, cognitive claustrophobia and negative ruminations.

Promoters of miracle diets are well aware of the overweight person's tendency to fix unrealistic weight-loss goals. Thus it is not surprising that they are so successful when they promise rapid weight loss, apparently obtained without effort. When the client becomes aware that the treatment has failed, he or she typically chucks out the diet prescribed, returns to old eating habits, and may even go on an eating binge to compensate for a useless and frustrating deprivation.

An approach adapted to your lifestyle with limited and realistic weight-loss goals and the opportunity to break certain eating rules on occasion will not only help you to prevent these reactions but also what Mahoney refers to as cognitive claustrophobia.

By curbing your eating behavior in order to lose weight rapidly, you build a "prison of absolutes" — this is my last piece of cake, I'll never eat French fries again, etc. — and cognitive claustrophobia results. The law of "all or nothing" which results from unrealistic standards intensifies your yearning for forbidden foods. As a matter of fact, a period of strict deprivation, in eating as in anything else, often creates an obsession with the desired object. Inevitably, you succumb to temptation and, in this case, eat your fill of what you want. Certainly, this eating behavior leads to enormous temporary relief but soon after it gives rise to feelings of guilt, failure and anxiety. That's a high price to pay for one small lapse. Then, because you've already ruined everything, why not take the day off? Usually, two or three days later, the dieter again puts on the yoke of over-strict limits. Then a new lapse occurs and the vicious circle continues.

Your role is to prevent and, as much as possible, eliminate this type of irrational idea, which is often responsible for continued weight increase and a feeling of impotence about your eating.

The third type of cognitive behavior which can obstruct the program's progress is negative rumination. The day after a certain kind of eating behavior, the person in treatment may silently repeat discouraging and self-disparaging statements such as: "I don't have any willpower," "I'll never succeed at anything," "I always fail," etc. As we can see, these remarks are vague and all-encompassing. It would be difficult to prove such assertions since a specific and often insignificant event has obviously been generalized to cover the entire personality.

To get a better idea of the effect of this inner monologue on behavior, imagine for a moment that a friend or colleague made the same comments to you. You would certainly react strongly. Of course, the emotional impact is less when you criticize yourself but it is important enough to subtly and progressively induce moods of depression which, in turn, will influence eating behavior in the manner described above.

From now on, you must proceed to eliminate any irrational ideas you may have and remain on guard during the treatment for when such ideas come up. Here is a brief plan of action:

1. Fix limited and realistic weight-loss goals. For the time being, think more of modifying your eating and physical habits as well as these inner monologues if you are subject to them.

2. Do not put absolute limits on your eating behavior; follow the program instead. Even if you lose only a little weight at the beginning, the weight loss will be gradual, continuous and lasting.

3. Be aware of all the self-destructive criticism you make, stop this behavior as soon as it begins and substitute, if possible, positive and encouraging behavior. To do this, immediately prepare some comments you can use deliberately such as: "I am more and more aware of the damage I am doing myself by being so self-critical," "I have enough control to stop this behavior," "I'm looking good today," etc. Write these sentences on the following lines. They will be useful in due course.

_____

_____

_____

_____

_____

_____

_____

_____

_____

_____

2. Get information on food intake and energy expenditure

a) Food intake

Overweight people are often well aware of the forbidden foods and the preferred foods in a strict diet. Everyone knows that chocolate is a high-calorie food and plain yogurt, a sensible substitute. However, experience shows that few people know the principles of a balanced diet. Re-education on eating is not only desirable but possible, and will increase the chances of the treatment's success.

The food-information section will help you better understand the rules of good eating and teach you to choose and prepare foods to get the maximum energy from them while minimizing your calorie intake.

Read it and you will probably be surprised at the changes you can make in your food intake.

b) Energy expenditure

We all know that the lack of activity in modern living should be paralleled by a reduction in the quantity of food we consume. Overweight people rarely make the necessary adjustment of exercising more and eating less.

Among the living habits associated with obesity, inactivity is undoubtedly the most important. It is rare that an obese person is intensely active physically : while overeating, the person walks very little or slowly, does not engage in strenuous exercise and generally leads a very sedentary life. The professional or social life may be very active but talking, writing or attending courses takes less energy than dancing, swimming or climbing stairs. Research has sufficiently shown the importance of physical activity in ensuring a general sense of well-being that it would be superfluous to explain the advantages of this strategy here.

In the exercise-information section, you will find all the relevant information for gradually changing your physical activity level. Did you know, for example, that a person normally eats less when he or she begins exercising? That the weight lost during an exercise-diet program is made up of 98% fat as compared to 75% for a diet without exercise? Being better informed can help you see the advisability of a different lifestyle.

3. Have the necessary information to respect the treatment's requirements

The preceding pages give a sufficiently detailed idea of the program for understanding the relative importance of the motivation factor. You can do it if you want to, but you only want to if you can as well. Wanting to lose weight is being able to solve this problem and having the information to do it. Now it's up to you.

DETAILED TREATMENT PROGRAM

ATTENTION!

If the preceding pages have not convinced you of the validity of this program, it would be better not to undertake it. In our opinion, you have to believe in the treatment if you are to meet one of the essential requirements for its success: systematically perform each exercise proposed.

Furthermore, we also believe that this task will be much easier if you begin the program at an opportune time. Choosing an exam period or spring-cleaning time or beginning while you are going through a difficult emotional or financial situation in your life will increase the risks of giving up or failing. And failure may affect your ability for self-control and reduce your motivation to try a new treatment some day.

If, in spite of all these cautions, you are still ready to commit yourself, follow the guide.

The program is spread out over ten weeks. This will give you time to acquire better control of your eating environment. As for your weight, it will have decreased and will continue to decrease after the end of the program if you follow the guidelines closely.

For each week of the program, we will fix goals and list different tasks to accomplish, while explaining them and supplying you with the necessary material.

FIRST WEEK

Objectives

1. Begin keeping a food-intake diary.
2. Follow the first rule.

1. Begin keeping a food-intake diary

The food-intake diary is your logbook for the first weeks of treatment. It will be your yardstick for measuring your eating behavior; it will supply you with all the necessary data for the problem-solving process. Therefore, you must make entries every day so that you can gather all useful information and make immediate evaluations.

The diary has seven sections:

a) **"Food section":**
Write down everything you eat or drink, except water.

b) **"Quantity" section:**
Write down the quantity (ounces, grams) or the volume (litre, ml.) of all food and drink consumed.

c) **"Time" section:**
Note the time of each meal or snack.

d) **"Exact place" section:**
Indicate the places where you eat as precisely as possible. For example, if you eat at home, specify the room.

e) **"Hunger" section:**
On a scale of one to five, assess the degree of hunger felt just before eating. If you were not hungry, put down 1 and if you were very hungry, put 5.

f) "Prevailing circumstances" section:

Indicate the circumstances which were dominant when you ate: what occurred just before eating (I just finished studying, I was watching television, I just got home, etc.) or something that was happening while you were eating (I was reading, I was watching television, there was a party, etc.) or something that happened after you ate (I had to go to work, I had to go out just after, someone was coming to visit, etc.). This way you can indicate the feeling you had while eating (disappointment, boredom, happiness, etc.). This section calls for special attention; it requires effort but it will give you a lot of information about your eating environment. Don't omit it!

g) "List of rules" section:

List the rules you followed during the day.

2. Follow the first rule: everything you eat, you eat while seated

From now on, you must sit down each time you eat, whether it be a meal, a snack or a dish you are checking for seasoning.

Sometimes it is difficult to make yourself sit down to eat, but by strictly following this rule you will discover its advantages. Experience teaches us that the difficulty of following a rule is often proportional to its usefulness.

Above all, do not begin a diet! The main objective of the treatment is not food as such but the eating environment. Fill in your diary carefully and follow the rule of the week.

Have a good week!

Material to use

FOOD-INTAKE DIARY

Day : _____

Food	Quantity	Time	Exact place	With whom	Hunger (1-5)	Prevailing circumstance

Make a list of the rules you have followed today :

SECOND WEEK

Prerequisites

1. Having kept a food-intake diary during the first week;
2. Having always eaten seated.

Objectives

1. Write the food-intake diary;
2. Follow the second rule;
3. Plan some rewards.

1. Write the food-intake diary

Continue to fill in your food-intake diary each day. From next week on, you will begin to analyze it in more detail. As this diary will differ from those preceding it, make 14 photocopies of the sample diary included.

2. Follow the second rule: always eat in an eating environment

An eating environment is a place specifically designed for consuming food. You may no longer eat in the living room, in your bedroom, in the street, in a car or on the subway. As you can see, your eating environment will be more restricted than it used to be.

Don't forget that the rules are cumulative, that is, this week you will always eat seated and always in an eating environment.

3. Plan some rewards.

So that the changes taking place will persist through the weeks to come, it is important that they be rewarded. Behavior that is rewarded has a greater chance of repeating itself and persisting than behavior followed by a negative consequence or just ignored.

From this week on, you should plan rewards for having followed your rules that day. The more closely the reward follows on the behavior, the more it will reinforce it. Also, as far as possible, you should plan rewards that are easily accessible throughout the day.

The rewards are divided into two main types: verbal rewards (I'm happy with myself, I followed my rules) and behavioral rewards (I listened to a little music to reward myself for following my rules). Behavioral rewards can satisfy physical and material needs or psychological needs (in the first case, I bought a dress and in the second, I called a friend).

You will undoubtedly notice that you are already using some rewards and that often they have to do with food (an ice-cream cone after working, for example). Let's look at behavior which can serve as rewards, putting aside eating gratification. Complete the following list:

LIST OF REWARDS

REWARDS

Behavioral		
Verbal	**Physical or material**	**Psychological**
Self-encouragement • I did a good job of following my rules • I have excellent control over my eating behavior • I'll probably succeed in this treatment if I continue to follow my rules	• Buying oneself small objects: magazines, newspapers • Wearing perfume • Using bath oil	• Taking a short rest • Telephoning a good friend • Putting off a chore that you don't want to do right away • Doing something pleasant that you don't often let yourself do

Remind yourself that a reward reinforces behavior only insofar as it follows it. For example, if you choose going to the movies as a reward, you can give yourself this treat only if you have followed your rules properly that day.

If you apply the planned reward without having respected the rules, you will increase the chances of this latter behavior (i.e. not following the rules) repeating itself.

To sum up:

a) Plan one or more rewards;

b) Apply the planned reward(s) **if you are respecting the rules**;

c) Do not reward yourself as planned if the rules have not been followed correctly.

Material

For the next two weeks, you should enter in your food-intake diary all the rewards you have given yourself each day. Use the following model for collecting this additional information.

Material to use

FOOD-INTAKE DIARY

Day : _____

Food	Quan-tity	Time	Exact place	With whom	Hunger (1-5)	Prevailing circunstance	Rewards

Make a list of the rules you have followed today :

THIRD WEEK

Prerequisites

1. Having kept a food-intake diary;
2. Having always eaten seated in an eating environment;
3. Having completed the list of rewards, given them during the week and entered them in the food-intake diary.

Objectives

1. Write the food-intake diary;
2. Follow the third rule;
3. Begin to make a list of distinct eating stimuli.

1. Write the food-intake diary

You will continue to write your food-intake diary carefully. Soon you will have to fill in another kind of diary.

2. Follow the third rule: eat without engaging in any other activity

From this week on, you will no longer be able to eat while doing something else such as reading, writing, watching television or doing the laundry. Of course, you can always talk, discuss or listen to music. But, for instance, if you have a tendency to have an aperitif while you are occupied with some other activity (preparing the meal, reading the paper), you will finish your drink before doing it.

3. Begin to make a list of distinct eating stimuli

Making a list of distinct eating stimuli will help you, first, to identify the factors that affect your food consumption and, second, to define your problem eating behavior methodically. In the weeks that follow, we will use the problem-solving process to bring about the changes desired.

From the food-intake diaries of the past weeks, you must begin to identify the problem eating structures, foods, times and places with the help of the list of distinct stimuli that you will find in the "Material to use" section.

Problem structures: this is the basic design of your eating behavior. The appropriate questions for drawing it up are as follows:

a) Do you eat three meals a day?

b) Do you have your meals at regular hours?

c) Is your food consumption spread out evenly in the day or do you eat more in the evening than in the morning, etc.?

d) Is there a reasonable time lapse between your meals (around five hours)?

e) Do you eat slowly (20 minutes or more)?

f) Do you leave the table after finishing the meal as such (a meal an hour long or less)?

When the answer to any of these questions is No, enter the problem structure in the column provided for this.

Problem foods: all foods that you don't know how to resist.

Problem times: the times of the day when you have more difficulty controlling your food consumption.

Problem places: all non-eating places where you eat and all eating places where you tend to eat in larger quantities or be less concerned about the quality of what you eat.

This stage of the treatment is important since it corresponds to the problem(s) definition stage. Be sure to carefully fill in the table below. The last two sections — social situations and prevailing circumstances — will be explained during the next week of treatment.

Material to use

LIST OF DISTINCT
EATING STIMULI

Structures	Foods	Times	Places	Social situations	Prevailing circumstances

FOURTH WEEK

Prerequisites

1. Having kept the food-intake diary;
2. Having always eaten seated in an eating environment and not engaged in any other activity;
3. Having given yourself rewards after respecting rules and entered them in the corresponding column of the food intake diary;
4. Having made a list of the distinct food stimuli previously described.

Objectives

1. Write a new food-intake diary;
2. Follow the fourth rule;
3. Complete the list of distinct eating stimuli;
4. Make a list of all problem eating behavior;
5. Read the first part of the Food section.

1. Write a new food-intake diary

From this week on, the food-intake diary changes format (see Material to use). You will no longer have to write down everything you eat. From now on, you will only note the behavior where you have not kept to the rules and exaggerated behavior, i.e. behavior where, although you followed the rules, your consumption posed a problem in terms of quantity or quality.

For these two types of behavior, the diary will indicate:

a) Antecedent: the activity you were engaged in just before eating;
b) Behavior: the food(s) you have consumed;
c) Reward(s) of eating behavior, that is the positive effect(s) of this behavior on your mood: e.g. diversion, relaxation, rest, etc.;
d) Alternative behavior: behavior you could have adopted in the place of eating behavior, behavior which would have given the same type of reward(s).

You should fill in this food-intake diary until the end of the treatment. It is particularly important to clearly identify the rewards for your behavior, first because they reinforce it and then because they often suggest possible alternative behavior. Make the copies needed of the sample diary which will follow.

2. Follow the fourth rule: take at least 20 minutes to eat a meal

From now on, you should take at least 20 minutes to eat a meal. Why 20 minutes? According to glucose regulation theories, it takes about 20 minutes from the time eating begins before the satiety centre located in the hypothalamus is stimulated.

Thus you can eat a lot of food in a very short time before feeling full when you eat, but then feel stuffed a few minutes later. If you take more than 20 minutes to eat, you will begin to feel full at the end of 20 minutes and you will not enjoy overeating as much.

The following methods can help you slow down your eating behavior; use them if necessary:

- take only one mouthful at a time
- wait until you have swallowed that before taking another
- use small utensils (e.g. a dessert fork)
- put down your utensil after each mouthful
- take smaller mouthfuls.

3. Complete the list of distinct eating stimuli

To complete the list of distinct food stimuli, the problem social situations and prevailing circumstances must be identified.

Problem social situations: social situations where you tend to eat more uncontrolledly or in larger quantities.

Problem prevailing circumstances: circumstances which affect your food consumption in terms of both quantity and quality. They may be emotional (boredom, disappointment, happiness, etc.) or behavioral (eating before or after a more or less pleasant activity; while preparing a meal, etc.).

4. Make a list of all problem eating behavior

With the preceding list completed, we are ready to define one or more behavioral targets. This task is intended to group the different stimuli identified in order to accentuate the links between them. By using the list of problem eating stimuli, the stimuli which interact in the same behavior can be grouped. Imagine that in your eating-behavior structure, there is a lot of time between lunch and dinner and towards the end of the afternoon you have a tendency to nibble at something when you get home; it is highly possible that the delay between lunch and dinner encourages you to nibble at the end of the afternoon.

Therefore, you must try to find all the probable links between the stimuli on the "blacklist." You must isolate the behavioral targets and, as you now know their characteristics, it will be easier for you to make the appropriate modifications. Make a list on the sheet provided (list of problem behaviors).

This task is obviously important in identifying and defining the main eating problems which create or maintain your excess weight. Give it your total attention.

5. Read the first part of the food section.

The food section is divided into two parts : information relating to the Canada Food Guide and information about calories. This week you should read the section on the food guide. Maybe you'll feel like modifying your eating habits but in your own way — no diet!

Do not forget your goal : controlling your eating environment.

Material to use

NEW FOOD-INTAKE DIARY

Antecedents	Behavior	Rewards	Alternative behavior

LIST OF PROBLEM-EATING
BEHAVIOR

1. _____

2. _____

3. _____

4. _____

5. _____

6. _____

7. _____

8. _____

9. _____

10. _____

FIFTH WEEK

Prerequisites

1. Having kept the new food-intake diary;
2. Having always eaten seated in an eating environment without being involved in any other activity while eating, and taken at least 20 minutes for each meal;
3. Having reinforced the habit of following rules by rewards;
4. Having completed the list of distinct eating stimuli;
5. Having made a list of all problem eating behavior;
6. Having read the first part of the food section:

Objectives

1. Write the new food-intake diary;
2. Substitute alternative behavior for problem behavior;
3. Follow the fifth rule;
4. Read the second part of the food section;
5. Learn to use the problem-solving technique;
6. Check if the food consumed meets the guidelines for a balanced diet.

1. Write the food-intake diary

You will continue to write the new food-intake diary, paying special attention to the rewards which come up and to alternative behavior.

2. Substitute alternative behavior for problem behavior

As much as possible, you should substitute the alternative behavior identified last week for problem behavior. You will then be able to judge its suitability and now make necessary modifications. In the same way, you will apply the alternative behavior of this week's diary as soon as the problem situation recurs.

3. Follow the fifth rule: eat at least three meals a day

From now on, you should eat at least three meals a day. This rule does not forbid snacks: it only specifies the minimum number of daily meals. We consider that an eating behavior is a meal when it includes at least three components: for example, a soup, a meat plate and a dessert, or juice, a piece of cheese and some bread are two possible menus. Don't forget that the meals must last at least 20 minutes.

4. Read the second part of the food section.

It is important to read the second part of the food section before using the problem-solving technique.

5. Learn to use the problem-solving technique

We have already introduced the problem-solving technique in six steps:
- defining the problem
- listing strategies or solutions
- analyzing the solutions
- choosing one or several strategies
- applying the chosen strategies
- evaluating the effectiveness of the strategies applied

With the help of this technique, we provide a solution to the problem eating behavior identified last week. But to master the technique, we will first choose typical problems: how to reduce sugar and saturated fat consumption and how to increase energy expenditure.

How to reduce sugar consumption?

Consult the sheet provided for this exercise (see Material to use). With the problem already defined, you must first list different strategies for solving it. We are proposing several; it's up to you to complete the list. Don't forget that at this stage, quantity takes precedence over quality: don't reject any idea; just list them.

Now you must evaluate the strategies on your list, taking into account their relevance, the time/money investment they require, their ease of application or any other criterion that will favour an appropriate choice. In the evaluation column, enter the result of your analysis using + or – signs.

This step completed, you must choose the strategies you will use. To do this, put all the strategies evaluated as positive in a numerical list (1, 2, 3, etc.).

In step 5, you proceed to apply the chosen strategies. First plan the different modes of application (shopping, timetable, schedules,etc.) and then apply the strategies according to the fixed program.

At the end of the week, make a list of the results obtained. This evaluation enables you to keep the most effective strategies or make the modifications needed for implementing them. If necessary, repeat the problem-solving process until you find one or more appropriate strategies, and use them in future.

Problems relating to saturated fats and energy expenditure will be solved over the next two weeks.

6. Check if the food consumed meets the guidelines for a balanced diet

Since you are now acquainted with the Canada Food Guide,this exercise will let you evaluate to what degree you eat the foods essential to a balanced diet. Over the next three weeks,you will write on the sheet provided (see Material) the number of portions from the food groups that you eat each day. For now, this is simply to gather data and not to make changes.

Material to use

PROBLEM-SOLVING PROCESS

Problem definition:	**How to reduce your sugar consumption.**	**Application:** (put down the number corresponding to the strategy used and to its mode of application)

Inventory of strategies	**Evaluation** (+ or –)	**Choice** (list strategies in order of choice)	Sunday: _____ Monday: _____ Tuesday: _____ Wednesday: _____ Thursday: _____ Friday: _____ Saturday: _____

Verification: enter the strategies which have proved effective.

1. Eat fruits
2. Make your own meals
3. Gradually reduce consumption
4. Stop buying sugar
5.
6.
7.
8.
9.
10.
11.
12.
13.

THE FOOD GROUPS IN YOUR DIET

	Sunday	Monday	Tuesday	Wednesday	Thursday	Friday	Saturday
Dairy products (at least 2 portions)							
Meat and substitutes (at least 2 portions)							
Fruits and vegetables (at least 3 to 5 portions)							
Bread and cereals (at least 3 to 5 portions)							

SIXTH WEEK

Prerequisites

1. Having kept the food-intake diary;
2. Having followed the first five rules;
3. Having reinforced the habit of following eating rules by certain rewards;
4. Having read all the food section;
5. Having learned the technique of solving problems related to reducing your sugar consumption;
6. Having verified, using the Canada Food Guide, if you are consuming the foods essential to a balanced diet.

Objectives

1. Write the food-intake diary;
2. Apply the sixth rule;
3. Practise the problem-solving technique;
4. Check if you are eating the foods essential to a balanced diet.
5. Gradually modify your eating behavior to meet the minimum requirements of the Canada Food Guide.

1. Write the food-intake diary

Continue to write the new food diary to gather more information in case it proves to be necessary.

2. Apply the sixth rule: leave some food on your plate

The sixth rule asks you to leave a small amount of food on your plate. This has a double objective: on one hand, you are desensitizing yourself to a childhood dictum, i.e. always having to finish what's on your plate if you want dessert or because of some moral principle; on the other hand, you learn to resist an immediately available food temptation. Do this once a day at the meal of your choice.

3. Practise the problem-solving technique

To increase your mastery of the problem-solving technique, we want you to apply it to an eating problem shared by many Canadians: over-consumption of saturated fats. In the sheet provided (see Material) you will find all the steps for this procedure. Some strategies are already mentioned, but don't hesitate to make an exhaustive and more personal list.

4. Check if you are eating the foods essential to a balanced diet

As you did last week, every day you must evaluate to what degree your eating conforms to the Canada Food Guide. On the sheet included, put down the number of portions that you consume daily in each of the Guide's four groups.

5. Gradually modify your eating behavior to meet the minimum requirements of the Canada Food Guide

While evaluating your food consumption according to the standards of the Canada Food Guide, you may notice certain gaps. For example, you may be eating only one portion of fruit or vegetables per day or no dairy products. These gaps must be filled. To help modify your tastes and habits, proceed in gradual steps. Begin with the foods you prefer : the guide offers several choices in each food group. For example, if you don't like milk, eat yogurt or milk-based soups or introduce the target foods three times a week at first, then increase the frequency of consumption little by little. If necessary, use the problem-solving technique to define the gaps or to find change strategies and apply them over a period of several months so that the acquired habits are maintained. Plan a change program here and now and begin to apply it right away.

As you see, we are not talking about exceeding the standards. Don't restrict your eating behavior ; instead, fill in the gaps.

Material to use

PROBLEM-SOLVING PROCESS

Problem definition:	**Decrease your consumption of saturated fats**	**Application:** write in the numbers corresponding to the stratégies that you will apply this week.

List of strategies | **Evaluation** (+ or –) | **Choice**

Sunday: _____

Monday: _____

Tuesday: _____

1. Eat less meat _____ _____

Wednesday: _____

2. Remove fat from meat before cooking

Thursday: _____

3. Eat more legumes (peas, beans, lentils, etc.) _____ _____

Friday: _____

Saturday: _____

4. Put more emphasis on eating vegetables _____ _____

5. Limit yourself to one meat meal a day _____ _____

Verification:
Write in the strategies which have proved suitable for you this week.

6. Eat fish more often _____ _____

7. _____ _____

8. _____ _____

9. _____ _____

10. _____ _____

11. _____ _____

12. _____ _____

THE FOOD GROUPS IN YOUR DIET

	Sunday	Monday	Tuesday	Wednesday	Thursday	Friday	Saturday
Dairy products (2 per day)							
Meat and substitutes (2 per day)							
Fruits and vegetables (4 to 5 per day)							
Bread and cereals (3 to 5 per day)							

SEVENTH WEEK

Prerequisites

1. Having kept the food-intake diary;
2. Having followed the first six rules;
3. Having reinforced the habit of following the eating rules by certain rewards;
4. Having practised the technique of solving problems related to reducing your consumption of saturated fats;
5. Having verified, using the Canada Food Guide, if you are consuming the foods essential to a balanced diet;
6. Having begun to modify your eating behavior to meet the minimum requirements of the Canada Food Guide.

Objectives

1. Write the food-intake diary;
2. Follow the seventh rule;
3. Read the section on energy expenditure;
4. Practise the problem-solving technique;
5. Verify if you are eating the foods essential to a balanced diet.

1. Write the food-intake diary

2. Follow the seventh rule: change the sequence of your meal components

For most people, a meal follows a certain order such as soup, a main dish, a dessert and a beverage. With the goal of reducing your sugar consumption, you should change the sequence of the items in your meals. From now, you will have your beverage after your main course and your dessert after your beverage. If you are not in the habit of having a beverage after your dessert, you can ignore this rule or start having a beverage between your main dish and dessert.

3. Read the section on energy expenditure

As obesity problems are usually associated with a sedentary life, changes in your lifestyle are not only desirable but necessary.

First, read the section on energy expenditure.

4. Practise the problem-solving technique

This week you will use the problem-solving technique to find ways to increase your energy expenditure. Find simple solutions which will easily fit into your daily life and substantially increase your energy expenditure during the day without requiring too large an investment of time or money. Above all, look for easily available methods such as climbing stairs instead of taking an elevator. Any exercise is suitable, even if it doesn't last very long. It's the total amount that counts...On the page provided, add as many strategies as possible to those we are suggesting.

5. Check if you are eating the foods essential to a balanced diet

Continue to evaluate your food intake using the minimum standards of the Food Guide.

Material to use

PROBLEM-SOLVING PROCESS

Problem definition:	**Increase your energy expenditure.**		**Application:** write the number corresponding to the strategies you will use this week. Sunday: _____ Monday: _____ Tuesday: _____ Wednesday: _____ Thursday: _____ Friday: _____ Saturday: _____
List of strategies	**Evaluation** (+ or –)	**Choice**	**Verification:** Write the strategies which have proved suitable for you this week.
1. Walk more			_____
2. Don't use stairs			_____
3. Enrol in a sports activity			_____
4. Go hiking			_____
5. Make love			_____
6. Go swimming			_____
7. Go cycling			_____
8.			_____
9.			_____
10.			_____
11.			_____
12.			_____
13.			_____
14.			_____
15.			_____
16.			_____
17.			_____
18.			_____
19.			_____

THE FOOD GROUPS IN YOUR DIET

	Sunday	Monday	Tuesday	Wednesday	Thursday	Friday	Saturday
Dairy products (2 per day)							
Bread and cereals (3 to 5 per day)							
Fruits and vegetables (4 to 5 per day)							
Meat and substitutes (2 per day)							

EIGHTH WEEK

Prerequisites

1. Having kept the food-intake diary;
2. Having followed the first seven rules;
3. Having reinforced the habit of following eating rules by certain rewards;
4. Having read the section on energy expenditure;
5. Having practised the technique of solving problems relating to increasing your energy expenditure;
6. Having checked, using the Canada Food Guide, if you are consuming the foods essential to a balanced diet.

Objectives

1. Write the food-intake diary;
2. Write your physical-activity diary;
3. Follow the eighth rule;
4. Practise the problem-solving technique.

1. Write the food-intake diary

2. Write your physical-activity diary

For the next three weeks, you should write a diary of your physical activities showing the following elements: day, activity(ies) practised, duration of each activity and caloric value. To find out the caloric value of an activity, simply consult the physical-exercise information section.

Don't mention all your daily activities, just the ones whose specific goal is additional energy expenditure.

Use the sample sheet included to make the photocopies you will need.

3. Follow the eighth rule: complete the sequence of your meals before taking a second helping

This rule is intended to decrease the size of your meals. From now on you can only take a second helping of any dish after having completed the whole meal. For example, if you want a second helping of the main course, first you should have your beverage, your dessert and another serving of whatever you ate before your main course, i.e. soup, salad, etc.

4. Practise the problem-solving technique

Now that you have a better mastery of the problem-solving technique, you can deal with the problems identified during the second week of the treatment. Proceed as follows:

    a) Eliminate the behavior which is no longer a problem for you. It may be that you no longer have behavioral problems to modify.

    b) Decide the order in which you will solve the behavioral problems which remain.

    c) Apply the problem-solving technique to one type of behavior at a time.

    d) If necessary, repeat the process until you have gained satisfactory control.

Material to use

PHYSICAL-ACTIVITY DIARY

Day	Activity	Duration	Caloric value

PROBLEM-SOLVING PROCESS

Problem definition _____

List of strategies	Evaluation (+ or −)	Choice	Application	Evaluation
1.				
2.				
3.				
4.				
5.				
6.				
7.				
8.				
9.				
10.				

NINTH WEEK

Prerequisites

1. Having kept the food-intake diary;
2. Having kept the physical-activity diary;
3. Having followed the first eight rules;
4. Having reinforced the habit of following the rules by certain rewards;
5. Having applied the problem-solving technique to problem eating behavior.

Objectives

1. Write the food-intake diary;
2. Write the physical-activity diary;
3. Follow the ninth rule;
4. Practise the problem-solving technique;
5. Increase energy expenditure.

1. Write the food-intake diary

2. Write the physical-activity diary

3. Follow the ninth rule: reverse the sequence of problem snacks

Often the negative side effects of certain foods are eliminated or controlled by other eating behavior. For example, a very sweet or very salty food is usually accompanied or followed by a beverage. This beverage largely eliminates the negative side effects of a food that is pleasant at the time of consumption. Thus a good way of reducing the attraction of such foods is to reverse the food-drink sequence.

From now on, with problem snacks, you will exclude beverages or have them before eating the food you choose (sweet, salty, sour, acid, etc.)

4. Practise the problem-solving technique

Continue to use the problem-solving technique to deal with problem eating behavior.

5. Increase energy expenditure

Analyzing the physical-activity diary will let you establish the average time devoted each week to physical exercise. If there have been no changes in your living habits over the preceding weeks or if the information gathered is unsatisfactory, it is essential to make a concerted effort to increase your energy expenditure. Revise the problem-solving process on this subject by setting more realistic goals such as enrolling in a physical-activity course lasting two hours a week or using up 200 calories a day by walking more. You will only develop better habits through constant practice, reinforced as needed by rewards.

TENTH WEEK

Prerequisites

1. Having kept the food-intake diary;
2. Having kept the physical-activity diary;
3. Having followed the first nine rules;
4. Having reinforced the habit of following eating rules by certain rewards;
5. Having applied the problem-solving technique to problem eating behavior;
6. Having increased energy expenditure.

Objectives

1. Write the food-intake diary;
2. Write the physical-activity diary;
3. Follow the tenth rule;
4. Practise the problem-solving technique.

1. Write the food-intake diary

2. Write the physical-activity diary

The diary will let you check the changes in your energy expenditure and gradually make the necessary corrections in this area.

3. Follow the tenth rule: give yourself a delay between the urge to eat and actually eating

The primary objective of eating behavior is not always to appease hunger and to nourish the body. Sometimes it has many different functions, such as easing anxiety or boredom, marking pauses in the day, etc. Thus it is not surprising that the eating response is often inappropriate. During a period of anxiety, an obese person may eat for reassurance. And as eating behavior only calms the distress temporarily, this can result in the creation of a new source of anxiety. The vicious circle is set up.

To help you find answers to these situations, you will have to follow the tenth and last rule of this treatment.

From now on, each time you feel like eating something and the primary objective is not to satisfy hunger, you should engage in a pleasant activity before going to eat. For example, when you are tired of studying, instead of going straight to the refrigerator for a little distraction, listen to music, have a shower or take a short rest. If you still want to eat after this delay, you can do so. Of course, the more the pleasant activity is appropriate to the situation, the more you increase your chances of satisfying the real need and thus avoid using food as a compensation.

AND THE TREATMENT CONTINUES...

We advise you to continue this treatment until you have reached your weight-loss goal. Don't forget to:

A) Follow the food-intake rules

1. Always eat seated.
2. In an eating environment.
3. Do not engage in any other activity while eating.
4. Have 3 meals a day.
5. Allow at least 20 minutes per meal.
6. Leave some food on your plate.
7. Change the sequence of your meal components.
8. Complete the sequence of the meal before taking any second helping.
9. Reverse the sequence of problem snacks.
10. Give yourself a delay between the urge to eat and actually eating.

B) Use the problem-solving technique in difficult situations

C) Fit physical activity into your daily life

INFORMATION :

FOOD

THE CANADA FOOD GUIDE

What do you have to eat to be "healthy"?
Eating well is easy!
Follow the guide...

The Canada Food Guide [1] is a model to enable you to choose your foods judiciously. It meets your daily nutritional needs as established by Canadian nutritional standards. To obtain more than the 50 nutritional elements needed every day, all you have to do is choose a large variety of foods from each group. The number and size of the portions are indicated in each case.

The guide classifies foods in four groups:
— milk and dairy products;
— bread and cereals;
— fruits and vegetables;
— meats and substitutes.

These groups are not interchangeable; they cannot be substituted for each other. Thus you cannot eliminate one group without depriving yourself of vital nutrients.

Here are all the groups in detail.

---

1. See following pages.

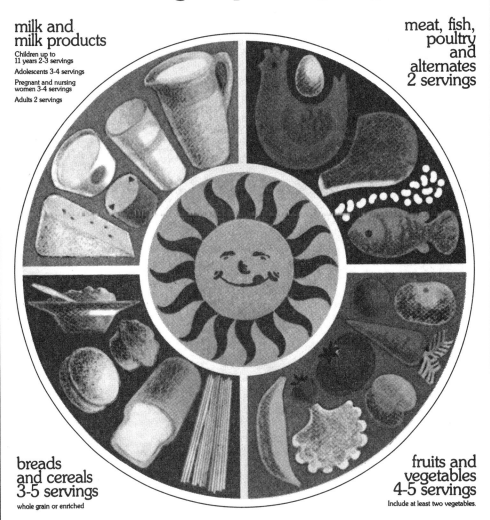

Canada's Food Guide

Eat a variety of foods from each group every day

milk and milk products
Children up to 11 years 2-3 servings
Adolescents 3-4 servings
Pregnant and nursing women 3-4 servings
Adults 2 servings

meat, fish, poultry and alternates 2 servings

breads and cereals 3-5 servings
whole grain or enriched

fruits and vegetables 4-5 servings
Include at least two vegetables.

Health and Welfare Canada   Santé et Bien-être social Canada   © Minister of Supply and Services Canada 1983
Cat. No. H59-32/1983-2E

Canada

Canada's Food Guide

Variety

Choose different kinds of foods from within each group in appropriate numbers of servings and portion sizes.

Energy Balance

Needs vary with age, sex and activity. Balance energy intake from foods with energy output from physical activity to control weight. Foods selected according to the Guide can supply 4000 – 6000 kJ (kilojoules) (1000 – 1400 kilocalories). For additional energy, increase the number and size of servings from the various food groups and/or add other foods.

Moderation

Select and prepare foods with limited amounts of fat, sugar and salt. If alcohol is consumed, use limited amounts.

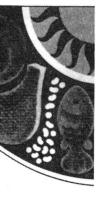

milk and milk products

Children up to 11 years	2-3 servings
Adolescents	3-4 servings
Pregnant and nursing women	3-4 servings
Adults	2 servings

Skim, 2%, whole, buttermilk, reconstituted dry or evaporated milk may be used as a beverage or as the main ingredient in other foods. Cheese may also be chosen.

Some examples of one serving
250 mL (1 cup) milk
175 mL (¾ cup) yoghurt
45 g (1½ ounces) cheddar or process cheese

In addition, a supplement of vitamin D is recommended when milk is consumed which does not contain added vitamin D.

meat, fish, poultry and alternates
2 servings

Some examples of one serving
60 to 90 g (2–3 ounces) cooked lean meat, fish, poultry or liver
60 mL (4 tablespoons) peanut butter
250 mL (1 cup) cooked dried peas, beans or lentils
125 mL (½ cup) nuts or seeds
60 g (2 ounces) cheddar cheese
125 mL (½ cup) cottage cheese
2 eggs

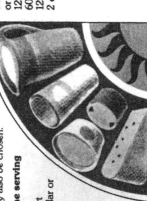

breads
and cereals
3-5 servings

whole grain or enriched. Whole grain
products are recommended.

Some examples of one serving
1 slice bread
125 mL (½ cup) cooked cereal
175 mL (¾ cup) ready-to-eat cereal
1 roll or muffin
125 to 175 mL (½ – ¾ cup) cooked
rice, macaroni, spaghetti or noodles
½ hamburger or wiener bun

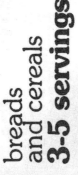

fruits and
vegetables
4-5 servings

Include at least two vegetables.

Choose a variety of both vegetables
and fruits — cooked, raw or their juices.
Include yellow, green or green leafy
vegetables.

Some examples of one serving
125 mL (½ cup) vegetables or fruits —
fresh, frozen or canned
125 mL (½ cup) juice — fresh,
frozen or canned
1 medium-sized potato, carrot,
tomato, peach, apple,
orange or banana

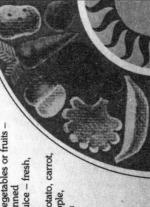

Milk and dairy products

Children up to 11 years old .... 2-3 portions
Teenagers .... 3-4 portions
Pregnant women
    and nursing mothers .... 3-4 portions
Adults: .... 2 portions

Examples of a portion:

250 ml. (1 cup) of milk (skimmed milk, buttermilk, powdered skim milk, partially skimmed milk, whole milk or evaporated milk).
250 ml. (1 cup) yogurt.
45 g. (1 1/2 ounces) cheddar cheese or processed cheese.

These recommendations are based on the calcium provision stipulated by Canadian nutritional standards. For the adult population, on the average, 80% of calcium needs are met by the milk and dairy products group. These products are also good sources of Vitamins D, A, B (especially riboflavin) and protein.

Other dairy products, such as butter, whipped cream, sour cream or cream cheeses, cannot be considered as equivalent portions in this group because of their high fat and low calcium content. However, ice cream (1/2 cup) represents 1/3 of a portion.

Milk may consumed as is or as an ingredient in other dishes, such as puddings, cream soups, milkshakes or eggnog.

Calories and dairy products

You can make a good choice among dairy products and at the same time reduce calories, fat and sugar:

— By using skimmed or partially skimmed (2%) milk instead of whole milk (3.5% fat). Skimmed milk contains 50% fewer calories than whole milk (powdered or liquid); it makes a good substitute for whole milk in most recipes containing milk: pudding, sauces, soups, etc.

— By choosing low-fat cheeses such as: creamed cottage cheese (4% fat) whole milk ricotta (13% fat) mozzarella from partially skimmed milk (16% fat) skimmed milk process cheese (6 to 7% fat) Most other cheeses contain more than 25% fat; it is better to choose firm cheeses than cream cheeses as the latter are not considered to be portions because of their low calcium content.

— By choosing plain yogurt and adding fresh or dried fruits, you reduce the amount of sugar compared to commercial fruit yogurt.

The following table gives you an idea of the calorie count for 100 mg. of calcium. The calorie count of foods differs considerably for the same nutritional value.

Calorie count per 100 mg. calcium

	calories/100 mg. calcium
skimmed milk	33
partially skimmed milk	42
whole milk.	55
processed cheese	56
cheddar cheese	55
cream soup	112
ice cream	131
fruit yogurt	73
plain yogurt	36
instant milk pudding	121

Calcium needs:
   women: 700 mg.
   men: 800 mg.
   pregnant women, nursing mothers: 1200 mg.

Milk and Vitamin D

There are few readily available sources of Vitamin D. Because of this, milk is enriched with Vitamin D following Canadian food and drug regulations. Commercial products such as yogurt, puddings and cheese do not contain Vitamin D.

An adult's daily Vitamin D needs are met by only 1 1/4 portion of milk or homemade milk-based foods. Here are some other sources of calcium for people who omit milk products from their diet: nuts, sardines, canned salmon, unshelled sesame seeds, broccoli and soy products. In some cases, calcium and Vitamin D supplements may be necessary.

Bread and cereals

---

3 TO 5 PORTIONS PER DAY

Whole-grain products are preferable.

Examples of a portion:

1 slice of enriched or whole-grain bread
125 to 250 ml. (1/2 to 1 cup) of cooked or ready-to-eat cereal
1 roll, biscuit or bran muffin
125 to 200 ml. (1/2 to 3/4 cup after cooking) rice, macaroni, spaghetti, noodles, etc.
1/2 hamburger bun

The food guide leaves you the choice of the number and size of portions; menus depend on individual preferences and caloric needs.

Iron and Vitamin B source

The bread and cereals group is an excellent source of iron and Vitamin B. Also, whole-grain bread and cereals increase the alimentary fibre content in our diet. Many "miracle" diets, for some bizarre reason, completely eliminate carbohydrates, which means no bread or cereals. Because of this, they are unacceptable.

The choice of foods in this group makes the midday meal more varied and attractive, especially if you have to take a lunch with you. Why not vary the type and form of bread? For example, use whole-wheat bread, pumpernickel bread, raisin bread and so on? It's also very simple to vary sandwich fillings. Add a salad, fruit and a glass of milk to your sandwich and you have a complete meal. A muffin, bun or croissant with cheese, raw vegetables and fruit is another example of a nutritious and quickly prepared lunch.

Enriching cereal products

In Canada cereal-products enrichment is regulated only in the case of flour; all white flour must be enriched with iron, thiamine, riboflavin and niacin. There is no obligatory enrichment of cereals and pasta, so you should read the label to see if the product has been enriched. It is also better to choose brown rice or steamed rice rather than pre-cooked rice (minute or instant rice). The latter has very little nutritional value.

Whole-grain cereals = alimentary fibres

Alimentary fibres are the cellulose residues from digestion of certain foods (whole grains, fruits, vegetables and legumes). These residues absorb a certain quantity of water and contribute to the volume of stool. Because of our "refined" diet, the volume of stools is reduced and thus they remain longer in the intestine. According to Burkitt (1970), they remain almost three times longer than when the diet is rich in fibre. This results in a increase in intestinal cancer which is very widespread in industrialized countries.

One certain fact is that a fibre-rich diet facilitates the work of the intestines and, by this, reduces problems such as constipation and diverticulitis. Whole-grain cereals and breads are high in fibre and should be preferred to refined products.

The many different kinds of cereal on the market can lead to confusion over choice. Here is a list of some whole-grain cereals whose added sugar content is not very high:

- *fibrous wheat* (Shredded Wheat, Shreddies, Muffets).
- *fibrous bran* (All-Bran, Bran Buds)
- *oatmeal* (rolled oats, quick-cooking oats). Oatmeal in instant packets is refined.
- *semolina* (Wheat Hearts).
- *wheat or bran flakes* (Bran Flakes, Pep).
- *whole-grain mixes* (Granola, Harvest Crunch). Homemade mixes can contain less sugar.

Natural bran: Bran is the natural coating and the fibrous part of grain kernels. It is used especially as an ingredient in bran muffins, biscuits or bread. It can also be added to cereal mixes such as granola.

Fruits and vegetables

---

4 TO 5 PORTIONS PER DAY

Include at least 2 vegetable portions.

Examples of a portion:

125 ml. (1/2 cup) of cooked vegetables or fruits or their juice
1 medium-sized potato, carrot, green pepper, tomato, peach, apple, orange or banana.

The food guide recommends eating at least two portions of vegetables each day to meet our Vitamin A needs. Yellow, orange and dark green vegetables are carotene sources. Carotene is a precursor of Vitamin A, which means it is transformed into Vitamin A in the body.

Fruits and vegetables make up an almost exclusive source of Vitamin C. Vitamin C is highly perishable. Here are some ways to preserve its taste and value:

- Cover and refrigerate juice after squeezing or after opening the container (Vitamin C oxidizes when exposed to air).
- Reduce Vitamin C loss in water by cooking foods in a small amount of boiling water.
- Oven or steam cooking also reduces Vitamin C loss in water.
- Taste, appearance and nutritional value are better preserved by freezing than by bottling or canning.

Fruits and vegetables are also important sources of iron. Green leafy vegetables, dried fruits and potatoes are especially rich in iron.

Fruit-flavored drinks (fruit drinks, fruit punch) cannot be considered as fruit portions: they contain nothing from the fruit except added Vitamin C. Frozen, sugar-free fruit juices (orange, grapefruit) are excellent buys.

It is better to eat fruits and vegetables raw because of the alimentary fibres they contain. In the same way, it is better to choose, as often as possible, a raw fruit or vegetable rather than fruit or vegetable juice.

Raw fruit is thirst-quenching; it contains a great deal of water.

Why not eat a fruit when you are thirsty?

Fruits are an excellent substitute for carbonated beverages or fruit-flavored crystals.

Good sources of Vitamin A
- carrots
- spinach
- sweet potatoes
- dried apricots
- broccoli
- squash

Good sources of Vitamin C
- citrus fruits
- Brussels sprouts
- cauliflower
- fresh or frozen strawberries
- vitaminized apple juice
- green peppers
- fresh tomatoes

Good sources of iron
- broccoli
- spinach
- potatoes
- raisins
- prunes

Meat and substitutes

2 PORTIONS PER DAY

Examples of a portion:

60 to 90 gm. (2 to 3 ounces after cooking) of lean meat, poultry, liver or fish (not counting skin, bones and fat)
60 ml. (4 tbsp) of peanut butter
250 ml. (1 cup after cooking) of dried beans, dried peas or lentils
80 to 250 ml. (1/3 to 1 cup) of nuts or seeds
60 gm. (2 ounces) of cheese
2 eggs

Notice the weight of the portions: 120 to 180 gm. (4 to 6 ounces) of lean meat, etc. per day. According to a national survey of Canadian eating habits, this is just over half the daily meat consumption (285 gm. or 9.5 oz) of men between 20 and 39 years old.

It is not necessary to eat so much meat. Our bad habits give us a surplus of 350 calories a day and an increased level of cholesterol and saturated fat in the blood. The idea that a big steak is healthy is a myth. It is not a nutritional necessity. Two daily portions of 60 to 90 gm. (2 to 3 ounces) each of lean meat or a substitute provide all the protein we need without counting the protein supplied by the other groups in the food guide.

Fat content and meat

One of the goals of the "Quebec Nutritional Policy" is to reduce fat content in our diet by 25%. And 40 to 45% of the fats ingested daily come from meat (among men and women between 20 and 39 years of age according to a Nutrition Canada survey). If we want to reduce the total fat content in our diet, meat is the primary target.

How to reduce consumption of fat from meat

- By making a better choice of meats, for example:
  — horsemeat, poultry and liver contain less fat than pork, beef or lamb.
  — buying less tender cuts of meat as well as lower-grade categories containing less fat.
    the fat content of ground beef is regulated. It is easier to make a choice when you know the fat content in the three categories offered:
    lean ground beef: 17% fat or less
    medium ground beef: 23% fat or less
    regular ground beef: 30% fat or less
  — removing all visible fat before grilling a steak eliminates half the calories.
  — restricting the use of processed meats: sausages, pressed meats, etc.

- By regularly adding fish to the menu. Even so-called "fatty" fish contain hardly more than 12% fat.

- By reducing the size of meat portions, you will obviously eat less fat. To do this, you can begin by using meat more often as an ingredient in a recipe: for example, macaroni, chicken with rice, salads, stuffed peppers, etc. By choosing these dishes, you certainly consume less meat than when you eat a steak, roast or chop and they are just as appetizing.

Vegetable source meat substitutes

At least 85% of Canadians between the ages of 12 and 65 eat beef every day.

Why such a habit? Let's be more imaginative.

A good way of varying the menu — and eating better — is to choose vegetable-source dishes based on meat substitutes such as legumes, nuts, seeds and grains.

These substitutes are very beneficial:

- they do not produce cholesterol. It is a well-known fact that high blood cholesterol is one of the risk factors in coronary disease;
- for the most part, they are rich in polyunsaturated fats. These help reduce blood cholesterol levels;
- they are rich in fibre;
- they let us prepare more economical meals.

Other meat substitutes

- *Cheese:*
  Cheese compares favorably with meat in terms of protein value but is a poor source of iron compared to other choices in this food group. If cheese shows up frequently in your meals as a protein source, it would be a good idea to accompany it with green vegetables and bread.

- *Eggs:*
  There is a lot of concern about the high cholesterol content of eggs. However, a normal person can eat 3 to 5 eggs a week without problems. By choosing among the foods suggested up to now in the food guide, our fat and cholesterol intake will remain quite moderate.

It is not necessary to turn vegetarian but introducing several meatless meals per week will ensure a better-balanced diet.

Combining vegetable proteins

The efficacy of animal or vegetable proteins depends on the simultaneous presence of eight essential amino acids, which must be assimilated in certain proportions to form proteins the body can use. Human milk serves as a reference point because it is the most complete protein, that is, the product with the maximum net protein use. Vegetable proteins are not complete when the three classes — legumes, nuts and seeds, and grains — are used separately. But by combining two of these classes, you get a good-quality protein. For this reason, in a meal which does not contain animal-source protein, you should use the following combinations :

LEGUMES + GRAINS
(e.g. pea soup + bread)

NUTS AND SEEDS + GRAINS
(e.g. peanut butter and bread)

LEGUMES + NUTS AND SEEDS
(e.g. mixed bean salad + walnuts)

Grains may also be combined with dairy products to obtain a better protein value.

The Food Guide and calories

Does the Food Guide meet our calorie needs?

According to the Food Guide, balanced menus supply between 1 000 and 1 400 calories a day. This is the minimum : you cannot eat less than 1 000 calories a day without depriving yourself of one or more essential nutrients. Most of us need more than 1 400 calories a day.

How to evaluate your energy needs

Energy needs vary a lot from one person to another. These variations are due to age, sex and activity levels. Because of the multiple factors which modify energy needs, it is often difficult to establish an individual's calorie needs precisely and it not generally necessary to do so.

According to Canadian standards set to conform to the needs of the average person within an age and sex group, men from 19 to 65 years old require 3 000 to 2 300 calories respectively and women from 19 to 65 years, 2 100 to 1 800 calories.

How to satisfy your energy needs

To make up the deficit between the 1 000 to 1 400 calories in the Food Guide's daily menus and your daily needs, the guide recommends increasing the quantities of food consumed in each of the groups or adding foods from other categories. To reach and maintain an ideal weight level, it is important to choose wisely.

Attention!

We know that a surplus or a deficit of 7 700 calories represents a gain or a loss of one kilogram. This decrease or increase in weight does not occur in one day. Miracle diets which promise speedy "melting" of extra weight do not tell us that this weight loss is mainly due to loss of water from the muscles and results from ingesting less than 1 000 or 800 calories a day.

Foods from "other" categories

The Food Guide does not specify that we need a certain quantity of sugar or fat to be in good health.

Sugar

You do not need to eat concentrated sugar to stay healthy. On the contrary, we should reduce our sugar consumption to avoid problems such as dental cavities, obesity and diabetes. The natural sugar contained in fruits, vegetables, milk, bread and cereals is sufficient for our needs. Almost everything we eat is, at least partially, transformed into sugar by the body as our energy needs require it.

Control our sugar consumption

We consume nearly 2 pounds of sugar per week and 65 % of this amount comes from commercially prepared products.

To control this better, read the list of ingredients on every label. Sugar occurs in several forms: sucrose, dextrose, honey, molasses, brown sugar, syrup, etc. The further down the sugar comes on the ingredient list, the less the product contains. Avoid very sugary products;

choose another brand or prepare the product yourself when the commercial equivalent does not meet your standards. By preparing your own foods, you can reduce the amount of refined sugar or replace it with dried fruits or spices.

Fat content

A moderate consumption of fat plays a vital role in nutrition. Oils and some margarines contain a polyunsaturated fatty acid which is essential to the body : linoleic acid. As well, fat helps the absorption of the fat-soluble vitamins A, D, E and K.

According to all present statistics, however, lipids make up too large a part of our total energy ration — around 40%. It would be better if a smaller number of our calories came from this source. Numerous studies indicate that such a high lipid intake can be hazardous to our health.

Which fats to choose

To help prevent cardiovascular illnesses, the Canadian Committee on diet and cardiovascular illnesses advises reducing total fat and cholesterol consumption and replacing some saturated fats with polyunsaturated fats.

Saturated fats are mainly of animal origin: meat, butter, lard, some shortenings, cream, whole-milk cheeses, etc.

Polyunsaturated fats are mainly of vegetable origin: sunflower oil, corn, walnuts and Brazil nuts, sunflower seeds, margarines that indicate the percentage of polyunsaturated fats on the label, etc. In the ingredient list, look for 50% or more liquid oil content.

The information contained in the food section is intended for everyone. However, we recommend that diabetics and people with elevated levels of cholesterol or triglycerides obtain fuller information from a dietitian or a doctor before making any modifications in their eating habits.

INFORMATION:

PHYSICAL EXERCISE

The role of physical exercise in weight control was minimized and even ridiculed for a long time by obesity specialists. Mayer (1968) was one of the first to assert that physical inactivity was one of the most important causes for the increase in the number of overweight people in western society. The need to integrate physical exercise into an obesity treatment program is now commonly recognized for several reasons. Let's look at some of them:

1. Obesity occurs when food consumption surpasses energy needs; the excess is stored in fatty tissue in the body.
2. Intensive physical conditioning brings about a reduction in fatty tissue and an increase in muscle tissue. In fact, several studies on the role of physical activity in weight loss did not prove a significant loss of weight. However, they did establish beyond a doubt that adipose tissue diminishes and is replaced by muscle. Thus there is a fat weight loss.
3. Intensive physical training permits significant loss of fatty tissue even without dietary restrictions and, consequently, an increase in muscle mass. For this reason, physical activity linked to better eating control is a very effective approach in obesity treatment.

4. Among animals as well as humans, the most overweight subjects are among the most sedentary. Moreover, even if the food consumption of some obese persons is often superior to that of non-obese subjects, obesity sometimes results basically from a lack of physical activity.

5. Weight loss resulting from a physical activity program does not only depend on the activity practised but also on the program followed. For example, in several studies, it was noticed that subjects enrolled in a jogging program lost fatty tissue when they participated four times a week but no longer lost it when they participated twice a week. On the other hand, when the exercise program was intensified, adipose tissue was reduced in both cases.

6. The possibility of losing fatty tissue in specific parts of the body through special exercises has never been clearly demonstrated. Generally, no matter what kind of exercise is practised, adipose tissue will diminish in the areas where it is located. Also, both general and localized exercises will significantly reduce adipose tissues in specific areas. Nonetheless, one of the reasons for favouring general exercise over localized exercise is that general exercise improves all the body's musculature while reducing the amount of adipose tissue wherever it is found.

In short, the golden rules are as follows:

- Exercise regularly.
- Fit physical exercise into your daily life.
- Engage in intensive physical exercise.

To make a better assessment of the energy used up in your daily activities, we are supplying a list of physical activities and the number of calories they burn (see following pages).

Energy expenditure
in sports and recreation activities

ACTIVITIES	CAL/HR	CAL/MIN
Badminton	400	6.66
Boxing	700	11.66
Baseball	350	5.83
Basketball	550	9.16
Canoeing (low-speed)	400	6.66
Canoeing (high-speed)	800	13.33
Boating (motor)	150	2.50
Bowling	250	4.16
Playing cards	25	0.42
Climbing calisthenics	500	8.33
Slow bicycling	300	5.00
Brisk bicycling	600	10.00
Croquet	250	4.16
Slow dancing	350	5.83
Fast dancing	600	10.00
Field hockey	500	8.33
Fishing (from a boat or dock)	150	2.50
Football	600	10.00
Golf	250	4.16
Handball	550	9.16
Horseback riding	250	4.16
Hunting	400	6.66
Jogging	600	10.00
Karate	600	10.00
Various activities in a seated position requiring little or no movement	50	0.83

ACTIVITIES	CAL/HR	CAL/MIN
Various activities done standing requiring some arm movements	150	2.50
Various activities in a seated position requiring energetic effort..	150	2.50
Motorcycling	150	2.50
Scooter	100	1.66
Slow piano-playing	75	1.25
Fast piano-playing with arm movements	125	2.08
Organ-playing using arms and legs	150	2.50
High-speed running	900	15.00
Singing	50	0.83
Speedskating	600	10.00
Recreational skating	400	6.66
Skiing	450	7.50
Squash	550	9.16
Soccer	650	10.83
Recreational swimming	400	6.66
Competition swimming	800	13.13
Softball	350	5.83
Singles tennis	50	7.50

Energy expenditure
in daily and domestic activities
(Men)

ACTIVITIES	CAL/HR	CAL/MIN
Activities in seated position requiring minimal arm effort	75	1.25
Activities in seated position requiring vigorous arm effort	175	2.916
Activities in standing position requiring minimal arm effort	125	2.08
Activities in standing position requiring moderate arm effort	225	3.75
Answering the telephone	50	0.83
Taking a bath	125	2.08
Sedentary work seated	100	1.66
Sedentary work standing	150	2.50
Bookkeeping	50	0.83
Light carpentry	225	3.75
Heavy carpentry	375	6.25
Dictation	50	0.83
Driving a car	50	0.83
Driving a truck	150	1.66
Driving a tractor	150	2.50
Dressing and undressing	75	1.25
Hammering	250	4.16
Recreational gardening	250	4.16
Professional gardening	400	6.64

Energy expenditure
for daily activities and housework
(Women)

ACTIVITIES	CAL/HR	CAL/MIN
Activities in seated position requiring minimal arm effort	50	0.83
Activities in seated position requiring vigorous arm effort	150	2.50
Activities in standing position requiring minimal arm effort	100	1.66
Activities in standing position requiring moderate arm effort	200	3.32
Answering the telephone	50	0.83
Taking a bath	100	1.66
Making a bed	300	5.00
Sedentary work seated	75	1.25
Sedentary work standing	125	2.08
Bookkeeping	50	0.83
Brushing teeth or hair	100	1.66
Daily dishwashing	75	1.25
Dishwashing: heavy articles at high speed	125	2.08
Dressing and undressing	50	0.83
Driving	50	0.83
Dusting furniture	150	2.50
Eating	50	0.83
Filing	200	3.32
Routine housework	100	1.66
Doubles tennis	350	5.83
Volleyball	350	5.83

ACTIVITIES	CAL/HR	CAL/MIN
Strolling	200	3.32
Brisk walking	300	5.00
Watching TV or seeing a movie	25	0.42
Wrestling	800	13.33
Knitting	50	0.83
Machine-washing small articles	200	3.32
Machine-washing large articles	250	4.16
Light waxing and polishing at regular speed	200	3.32
Light waxing and polishing at high speed	250	4.16
Routine floor-sweeping	200	3.32
Vigorous, rapid floor-sweeping	300	5.00
Routine cooking	100	1.66
Rapid cooking	150	2.50
Reading	25	0.42
Routine floor-scrubbing	200	3.32
Vigorous, rapid floor-scrubbing	300	5.00
Sewing	50	0.83
Taking dictation	50	0.83
Typing	50	0.83
Climbing and descending	800	13.33
Writing	50	0.83

CONCLUSION:

THE MAINTENANCE PHASE

If you have followed the program, it is now several months later and you have lost several pounds and are in better health. You are also more skilled at solving your eating problems.

The skills you have acquired are guarantees that you will maintain your present physical shape. Obviously, you may still gain some weight. We live in a society that encourages being overweight: the food industry, social customs and automation of work continually create conditions that encourage us to overeat often unhealthy foods and lead sedentary lives. Of course, now you have better eating and physical-exercise habits as part of your lifestyle. But it would be unrealistic to believe that your weight will not change along with the changes that occur in your life. For example, as you age, your body burns fewer calories. You will then realize the importance of the skills you have acquired. Self-management is not a temporary project but a way of life. If the need arises, you can always use the problem-solving process to make necessary adjustments.

As long as you maintain a self-management mindset, variations in your weight will not plunge you into fits of frustration, depression or resignation. You know that your weight will undergo changes but you also know that you possess the skills for making the modifications needed.

With this in mind, we recommend the following techniques when you have reached your desired weight and are entering the maintenance phase.

1. **Don't worry about your weight.** You now control this area of your life. You are a new person physically and psychologically. You can now have confidence in yourself and in the skills you possess for managing your eating behavior. Let the era where you set strict limits for yourself and were obsessed with food, weight and diet questions be finished forever! All your attention should now be focused on maintaining your self- management skills.

2. If you want to, you can **gradually** abandon all the rules for restricting the eating environment which have been useful to you for acquiring or for maintaining the habits necessary to the changes desired. If, on the other hand, you enjoy these structures, you can certainly keep them as long as you wish. Remind yourself that you manage your life : if you lose certain habits with time, you know what to do to develop them again.

3. Weigh yourself once a month, never more. If there is a sudden increase or a continued increase from one month to another, you will certainly want to remedy the problem by evaluating the factors responsible for the change in your physical, social or intimate life.

4. Be creative in your solutions. It is dangerous to maintain a solution that works but is boring and difficult, because with time you will abandon it and lose all motivation for solving your problem.

5. Anticipate problems before they come up. For example, if you know that you usually gain weight on vacation, you can plan a new program of physical exercise or change some circumstances of your vacation project so that you can enjoy the good food you'll be treating yourself to while you're away.

Perhaps you feel you've learned nothing new from our recommendations and that, all considered, you feel responsible enough for your life now to solve problems when they come up. If so, our program has been a success.

We would appreciate your comments, no matter what results you have had. Send them to us at the following address:

Obesity Program
Psychological Guidance and Consultation Service
University of Montreal
2101 Blvd. Édouard-Montpetit
Montréal (Québec)
I I3C 3J7

Bibliography

Diet

BURKITT, D. Economic development, not all bonus. *Nutrition today.* **11**, 1, January-February 1977.

Le manuel du guide alimentaire canadien. Ottawa : Health and Welfare, 1977.

LAMBERT-LAGACÉ, Louise. *Menus de santé.* Montréal : Éditions de l'homme, 1977.

Nutrition Canada, Rapport sur les habitudes alimentaires. Ottawa : Health and Welfare, 1975.

Nutrition Canada, Résultats du Québec. Ottawa : Health and Welfare, 1975.

Rapport du Comité sur le régime alimentaire et les maladies cardio-vasculaires. Ottawa : Health and Welfare, 1977.

Standards de nutrition au Canada. Ottawa : Health and Welfare, 1975.

Une politique québécoise en matière de nutrition. Ottawa : Social Affairs, 1977.

Energy Expenditure

BOUCHARD, C., LANDRY, F., BRUNELLE, J., GODBOUT, P., *La condition physique et le bien-être*. Québec : Éditions du Pélican, 1974.

CLARKE, H. H., *Physical Fitness*, Research Digest, Série 5, No 2, 1975.

MAYER, J., *Overweight, causes, cost and control*, Englewood Cliffs, New Jersey : Prentice Hall Inc., 1968.

Eating behavior, self-management

ABRAMSON, E. E., *Behavioral approaches to weight control*. New York : Springer publishing, Co., 1977.

BRUCH, Hilde. *Eating disorders : anorexia nervosa and the person within*. New York : Basic Books, 1973.

FERSTER, C.B. *et al.* The control of eating. *Journal of mathematics,* **1**, 87–109, 1962.

MAHONEY, M. J., MAHONEY, Kathryn. *Permanent weight control*. New York : W. W. W. Norton et Co., 1976.

STUART, B. R., DAVIS, B. *Slim chance in a fat world.* Campaign, Illinois : Research press, 1972.

STUNKARD, A. *The pain of obesity*. New York : Plenum, 1976.